20-minute fitness

JAMES NEVELLI

THIS BOOK IS DEDICATED TO MY DEAR DAUGHTERS WHO ARE MY BACKBONE AND STRENGTH

Acknowledgments

I thank God for all the graces and blessings and for guiding me to write this book. A special thanks to all my family, trainers, clients, and students, especially those who exercised with me, trusting me with their lives and inspiring me to write this book.

Finally, I thank all my mentors for their guidance and support, which made this possible.

Thank you, everyone.

DISCLAIMER

We advise the reader to seek the medical advice of a Physician, Wellness Coach, and Nutritionist before engaging in any exercise, diet, or therapy program mentioned in the book.

The exercises and advice are for healthy individuals with no chronic disorders or health issues. We advise caution and request that you stop exercising if you experience any discomfort.

The writer or any entity associated with the book is not liable and will not be held responsible for any injury that may occur because of following any advice, exercise, or guidelines given in the book.

In witness whereof, the reader having read and understood the above does hereby voluntarily set his or her hand.

CONTENTS

CHAPTER 1.

INTRODUCTION: The Starting Point

Dear, even though there is an awareness of the need to exercise we are always skeptical about how to go about achieving our fitness goals and what exercise program is best suited to our body and our requirements. The question is no longer "to exercise or not to exercise" but how much, how often and with what intensity to exercise to confer maximum benefits in the promotion of well-being and fitness even when we have a limited amount of time in our busy schedule. If this is You, then this book is for You

Being a Fitness Professional, a Life Coach for the last 22 years, and an Acupuncture Therapist for the last 2 years, I've had the opportunity to interact with all types of people, I've seen the change in both the outward appearances and better outlook to life of both my clients and students after counselling and training. These are my findings:

Three to six months of consistent exercise with simple diet alterations and a positive attitude and mindset can give a person tremendous physiological and physical benefits. A few of the main physical changes that I have seen are Reduction of obesity, Rectification of Posture, Body sculpting, increase in bone density, control and reduction of osteoporosis, Control and reduction in arthritis, Control and relief from osteoarthritis, Lower cholesterol levels, control and reversal of blood pressure, reduces risk of coronary artery disease, reduces risk of cancer, controls diabetes, increased energy levels.

I have noticed that, along with a change in the body, the mind gets healed and perception changes. Within two to three weeks of starting a fitness program the psychology of the person too becomes more positive. Exercise develops a healthy body image and self-esteem. My students have gained optimum wellness, reduced depression, reduced anxiety, increased self-esteem and confidence, reduced stress levels, become more alert, and found themselves in a more positive mood with ample energy. For ladies having issues with PCOD, fibroids, or conceiving a child, I've found that if they lose an initial 3 to 5 kgs of body weight which reduces the fat in the tubes, this reduces the effects of PCOD, their chances of getting pregnant increased and I am blessed to know that so many of them have beautiful healthy babies now.

WHAT TO DO IF YOU DON'T LIKE EXERCISING?

In the fast-paced world of today, where juggling work, family, and personal time can feel overwhelming, finding ways to integrate physical activity into your daily routine is not just beneficial, it's essential. But, if you are one of those who somehow don't like the idea of joining an exercise routine and feel it's not your cup of tea, I've known people who are healthy and happy even with moderate daily physical activity which can be done around the house. Some of my acquaintances have made themselves healthier and more active by following a few of the below guidelines which have kept them generally fit.

You can start doing at least one of the activities listed below or combine activities for 30 minutes most days of the week, preferably daily. You can look for similar or additional activities in your surroundings to create an opportunity to enjoy maintaining and improving your quality of life.

Imagine transforming mundane tasks into opportunities for movement: opt for a brisk walk instead of a drive, take the stairs rather than the elevator, or get off the bus a few stops early to enjoy a refreshing stroll. Even activities like gardening, cleaning, and playing with children can double as effective workouts, burning approximately 150 calories per day or 1,000 calories a week. For instance, washing your car or tackling household chores for just 45-60 minutes can yield substantial calorie burn, while a simple 10-minute walk can rejuvenate your day. Remember, the more you weigh, the faster you'll burn calories, which can be a powerful motivator. By making these small adjustments, you'll not only boost your physical health but also enhance your mental well-being, creating a balanced lifestyle that empowers you to thrive. Embrace the movement—your body and mind will thank you!

The less vigorous the activity, the more time is needed to achieve health benefits. If you calculate the expending of calories, you will be surprised that the heavier you are the quicker you will burn calories initially. That is a great motivation for you to start if you are a bit on the heavy side. I've given you a table below where you can see how according to your weight you will burn calories.

Activity	Kcal/min/kg	55kgs	75kgs	95kgs
Walking normal pace	0.080	4.4	6.0	7.6
Sitting quietly	0.021	1.2	1.5	2.0
Cycling: @ 5.5 mph	0.064	3.5	4.8	6.0
@ 9.4 mph	0.100	5.5	7.5	9.5
Running: @11.5 min/mile	0.135	7.40	10.1	12.8
@8.0 min/mile	0.208	11.40	15.6	19.8

Adapted from McArdle WD, Katch FI, Katch VL. Exercise Physiology: Energy, Nutrition, and Human Performance. Philadelphia, Pa: Lee and Febiger; 1981.

Making simple dietary changes can significantly enhance your health and support your fitness goals, especially for busy women on the go. Start by embracing a variety of foods, ensuring you get all the essential proteins, vitamins, and minerals your body craves for balance. Aim for moderate protein intake from low-fat sources, and don't forget to prioritize your calcium needs for strong bones. When you're active, boost your carbohydrate consumption to make up 55-60% of your total daily calories, providing you with the energy needed for workouts and daily tasks. Reduce your carbohydrates if you lead a sedentary lifestyle as carbohydrates are for energy which transforms to fat if not utilized. If you need more muscle and bone strength, protein intake at approximately 20 to 30% is usually appropriate.

To optimize your nutrition, consider reducing your intake of alcohol, sugary drinks, and indulgent milkshakes. Instead, focus on hydrating with water or herbal teas. It's also wise to limit sodium to no more than 2,400 mg per day—opting for healthier alternatives like Celtic salt and Himalayan salt. Keep dietary fat at 30% or less of your total calories, and aim for less than 300 mg of cholesterol each day. By incorporating these straightforward adjustments into your lifestyle, you can create a nutritious and balanced diet that fuels your body and empowers you to achieve your goals!

Check out this ancient Chinese Body clock which has been used for centuries and still holds good even today. It shows you at what time each organ is working at its optimum.

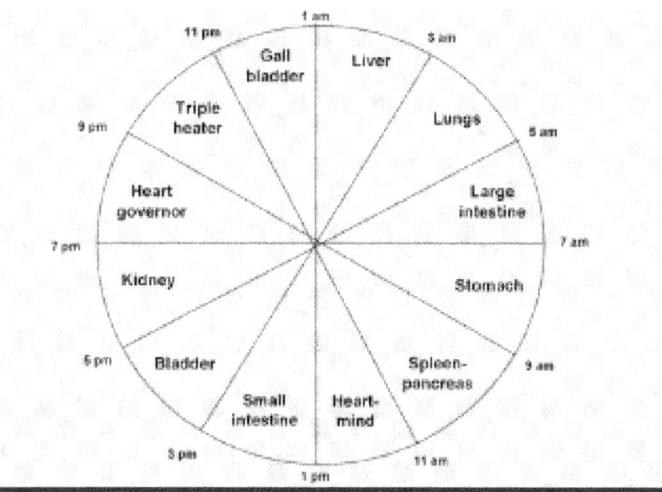

Chinese Body Clock: About, Benefits, Research

You may have heard of the body's biological clock before, but what about the Chinese body clock?

Rooted in traditional Chinese medicine, the Chinese body clock is based on the idea that you can make the most of your energy and specific organs by using them when they're at their peak.

The peaks of individual organs within the body vary. For example, the lungs are at their height between 3 a.m. and 5 a.m. every day.

But does this mean you should be up at the crack of dawn to make the most of these organs by exercising? Are there any significant advantages to prescribing the theories behind the Chinese body clock?

In this article, we'll take a closer look at this concept, why it's believed to be beneficial, and what the research says.

What's the Chinese body clock?

To understand the Chinese body clock, you first need to grasp the concept of qi or energy. In short, qi is a word used in Chinese medicine to describe energy. It consists of energy in every sense of the word. For example, Earth has qi, as does your body, and even thought and emotion.

It's also important to understand that energy is in a constant state of flux. It's continuously transforming as it moves within the body or between people and objects.

The Chinese body clock is built on the concept of qi or energy which is in a constant state of flux. So every day for each 24 hours, the electronic energy produced by the body moves in 2-hour intervals throughout the organ systems giving more preference to check out the functioning, restoring, and cleansing of those organs. While you're sleeping, this same energy draws inward to fully restore your body.

One of the most important 2-hour intervals is between 1 a.m. and 3 a.m., which is when the liver is believed to be cleansing the blood. It's during this time frame that the body begins to prepare for qi or purified blood and energy to move outward from the body again.

This table shows which organs correlate to the 2-hour intervals of the Chinese body clock.

2-hour interval	Organ and peak functionality
3–5 a.m.	**Lung:** This period is when the lungs are at their peak energy. It is believed to be an ideal time to exercise, as opposed to later in the day.
5–7 a.m.	**Large intestine:** This period is thought to be when you should give yourself enough time to honor the elimination function of the large intestine.
9–11 a.m.	**Spleen:** The <u>spleen</u> is thought to be <u>linked</u> to the stomach, which is in charge of receiving food and drink before ultimately fermenting them. During this period, it's believed that qi is being propelled upward by the spleen.
11–1 p.m.	**Heart:** Because the heart <u>represents peacefulness,</u> it's essential to reduce stress during this period, according to those who prescribe to the Chinese body clock.
1–3 p.m.	**Small intestine:** Heavier meals are believed to be more tolerated during this period, as the qi expands and begins to crest at midday.

3–5
p.m.

Bladder/kidney: It's believed that the **kidney** is in charge of containing qi, and it's **directly connected** with the bladder. Together, they excrete unwanted waste materials within the body.

7–9
p.m.

Pericardium: The **pericardium** is believed to be the **protector of the heart.** This period is when qi is supposedly regulated to prevent symptoms, such as nausea and vomiting.

9–11
p.m.

Triple burner: The triple burner refers to the organ system **as a whole,** and this period is thought to be when it generates the most amount of heat.

1–3
a.m.

Liver: Those who prescribe the Chinese body clock believe it's important to give your **liver** as little to process as possible during this period so it can focus on its several cleansing functions. This means eating your last meal of the day early and making sure it's light.

How can you use the clock to benefit your health?

By embracing the concept of the Chinese body clock, it's believed that you can potentially make the most of your specific organs and bodily functions when they're at their peak.

For example, according to the Chinese body clock, the lungs peak between 3 a.m. and 5 a.m. Getting up early for a morning exercise during this time may help you maximize the potential of these organs.

Guidelines for your exercise program.

 A well-rounded fitness program should aim to improve and maintain key components of health and fitness, such as **cardiorespiratory fitness, muscular strength and endurance, flexibility, body composition, and skill-related components.** As you get fitter through regular exercise you will realize that you are not only getting physically stronger but also feeling stronger as an individual in your thoughts and your soul. Become consistent with at least **5** days of a workout regime and then you can gradually increase the intensity of your workouts. This helps reduce the risk of injury and improves cardiovascular health. Regular exercise becomes a part of your life, enhancing both your physical and mental well-being. These benefits are available to everyone, regardless of age, with consistent, moderate exercise.

 While it's best to exercise under the guidance of a certified trainer, there are some tips to help you work out safely and effectively by yourself. First, ensure your **alignment, form**, and **stabilization** are correct throughout the exercise. Avoid stressing weak areas of your body by moving smoothly and taking short breaks between exercises, especially in the first month. Perform exercises with a comfortable range of motion and speed. *Always check and maintain your posture* - shoulders square, back straight, abdomen slightly tucked in, and feet hip-width apart. Using a mirror can help ensure correct posture. Make sure the exercises you do are suitable for your body. If you have any existing conditions like back issues or knee pain, address these first. For chronic conditions like diabetes or high blood pressure, start with stretching exercises for the first three months before moving on to more intense workouts.

 It's important to listen to your body during exercise. Pay attention to how your body feels, take breaks, and hydrate as needed. **Room temperature water is the best hydrant**. Have a sip or two when required. Maintain a steady breathing pattern—inhale and exhale with each movement. Keeping your posture in check throughout your workout helps avoid injuries and maximizes effectiveness. The rest periods between each exercise can initially be 10 to 20 seconds and as the months go by you can reduce or eliminate it. Your body temperature should *gradually rise* at the beginning of a workout and *gradually relax* at the end. So a minimum of 5 minutes of warmup and stretches are essential at the beginning and end of each workout regime. By following these guidelines, you can enjoy a safe and effective workout routine that enhances your overall health and fitness. Remember, ***consistency is key,*** and it's important to listen to your body and adjust your routine as needed.

CHAPTER 2

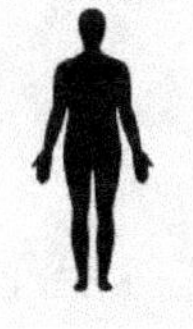

THE READINESS QUIZ

If you are a beginner and a first-time exerciser it is essential that you check if you are ready in mind and body to start a workout program. ***Are you ready to change your life today?*** I have put together a readiness quiz for you to ask yourself.

Now that you are ready to be you, to get fit, tone and sculpt your body, get clarity in thought, lose excess weight, be more active, feel energized, be happy, and feel fulfilled in life, please take this Exercise and Life change Readiness Quiz to learn if you need to make any attitude adjustments before you begin to ensure success in your program. Answer true or false to each of the below statements. It's important to be honest as these answers reflect the way you really are, not how you would like to be.

Answer True or False

1. I have thought a lot about my eating habits and physical activities to pinpoint what I need to change.

2. I have accepted the idea that I need to make permanent, not temporary, changes in my lifestyle, eating, and activities to be successful.

3. I will only feel successful if I lose a lot of weight or have massive inch loss.

4. I accept the idea that it's best if I tone up and lose weight slowly.

5. I'm thinking of toning my body and losing weight now because I really want to, not because someone else thinks I should.

6. I think losing a few inches and losing weight will solve other problems in my life.

7. I am willing and able to increase my regular physical activity.

8. I can follow the exercise and new food habits routine successfully if I have no "slip-ups".

9. I am ready to commit some time and effort each week to organizing and planning my food and activity programs.

10. Once I lose some inches and initial weight, I usually lose the motivation to keep going until I reach my goal.

11. I want to start an exercise program, even though my life is unusually stressful right now.

B. Some thought-provoking questions are; How will a healthy lifestyle complement or support this? What do you hope to get out of this experience?

Make a note of your goals, and how much toning, inch loss, or weight you wish to lose in a particular time frame say three three-month or six-month period. What habits are you going to change in food, attitude, and lifestyle? Make a note of what you feel you can accomplish if all things work in your favor. What do you really want? Think again, what are you willing to change to reach your goal? "Where do you feel you are now on this journey? Do you consider yourself a fit and healthy person; How is your level of fitness? What food do you keep around the house and what are your food habits? In your daily food intake, what is the approximate quantity, quality, and ratio of carbohydrates, protein, and fats? Are your sleep habits good? Do you get at least 6 to 7 hours of deep sleep to rest your mind and body? What is the balance of your work-home routine, at this point?

What are the obstacles you may face? What could stop you from moving forward? How will you overcome this? What if they were removed? How would that change the situation? What are the pros and cons of this option?

How can you keep yourself motivated? What support do you need?

Now that you know your strengths and weaknesses you can work on how you can make the necessary changes with the help of a family member, friend, or mentor. This will ensure you can stick with the program in all circumstances.

You need to be true to yourself in answering all the questions and congratulate yourself when you change. Now go ahead and answer the questions given below to make sure your physical state is appropriate to follow an exercise program.

C. PAR-Q

(Physical Activity Report-Questionnaire)

Please read the questions carefully and answer each one honestly: Yes or No.

1. Has your doctor ever said that you have a heart condition and that you should only do physical activity recommended by a doctor?

2. Do you feel pain in your chest when you do physical activity?

3. In the past month, have you had chest pain when you were not doing physical activity?

4. Do you lose your balance because of dizziness, or do you ever lose consciousness?

5. Do you have a bone or joint problem (for example, back, knee, or hip) that could be made worse by a change in your physical activity?

6. Is your doctor currently prescribing drugs (for example, water pills) for your blood pressure or heart condition?

7. Do you know of any other reason why you should not do physical activity?

If you answered "Yes" to one or more questions:

Talk with your doctor by phone or in person BEFORE you start becoming much more physically active and BEFORE you embark on this beautiful new journey.

If you answered "No" to all questions:

If you answered "No" honestly to all PAR-Q questions, you can be reasonably sure that you can start your exercise and life-changing program.

Your next step will be your physical fitness appraisal– this is an excellent way to determine your basic fitness to plan the best way to live actively.

It is also highly recommended that you have your blood pressure evaluated. If your reading is over 144/94, talk with your doctor before you start becoming much more physically active.

Please note: If your health changes so that you then answer "Yes" to any of the above questions please check with your doctor before resuming any program.

CHAPTER 3

FORM, TECHNIQUE AND BREATHING

By following these guidelines, you'll be well on your way to a safe and effective workout routine.

JUMPING JACKS

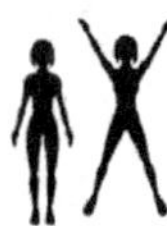 **How to Perform Jumping Jacks**

1. *Starting Position*: Stand upright with your feet together and your arms at your sides.
2. *Jump and Spread*: Jump up and spread your legs out to the sides while simultaneously raising your arms above your head. Your body should form an "X" shape at the peak of the jump.
3. *Return to Starting Position*: Jump again and bring your legs back together while lowering your arms to your sides. Return to the starting position and repeat.

Breathing Technique: Inhale as you jump and spread your legs and arms. Exhale as you return to the starting position.

Tips for Proper Form:

- *Controlled Movements*: Perform the exercise in a controlled manner to maintain balance.

- *Soft Landings:* Land softly on the balls of your feet to reduce impact on your joints.

- *Engage Core:* Keep your core engaged to maintain stability.

Common Mistakes to Avoid

- *Hard Landings:* Avoid landing heavily on your feet to prevent joint strain.

- *Flailing Arms:* Keep your arm movements controlled and coordinated with your leg movements.

- *Inconsistent Breathing:* Maintain a steady breathing pattern to ensure adequate oxygen flow.

LUNGES

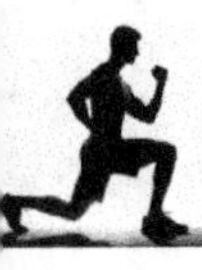

How to Perform Lunges

1. *Starting Position:* Stand upright with your feet hip-width apart. Keep your hands on your hips or by your sides for balance.
2. *Step Forward:* Take a big step forward with your right foot. Ensure your torso remains upright and your shoulders are back.
3. *Lower Your Body:* Lower your body until your right thigh is parallel to the ground and your right knee is directly above your ankle. Your left knee should hover just above the floor, forming a 90-degree angle with your left leg.
4. *Push Back Up:* Push through your right heel to return to the starting position. Repeat the movement with your left leg.

Breathing Technique: Inhale as you step forward and lower your body. Exhale as you push back up to the starting position.

Tips for Proper Form

- *Knee Alignment:* Ensure your front knee does not extend past your toes to avoid strain.

- *Torso Position:* Keep your torso upright and avoid leaning forward.

- *Controlled Movements:* Perform the exercise in a slow and controlled manner to maintain balance and engage the muscles effectively.

Common Mistakes to Avoid

- *Overstepping:* Taking too large a step can cause imbalance.

- *Knee Position:* Allowing the front knee to go past the toes can lead to knee strain.

- *Leaning Forward:* This can put unnecessary stress on your lower back.

SQUATS

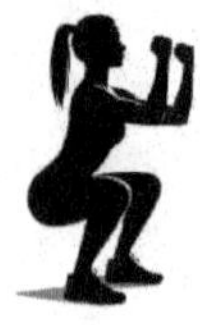

How to Perform Squats

1. *Starting Position:* Stand with your feet shoulder-width apart. Keep your toes slightly pointed outwards. Hold your hands out in front of you for balance or place them on your hips.
2. *Lower Your Body:* Engage your core and keep your chest up. Push your hips back as if you are sitting in a chair. Bend your knees and lower your body until your thighs are parallel to the ground. Ensure your knees are tracking over your toes and not caving inward.
3. *Return to Starting Position:* Push through your heels to stand back up. Squeeze your glutes at the top of the movement.

Breathing Technique: Inhale as you lower your body into the squat. Exhale as you push back up to the starting position.

Tips for Proper Form

- *Knee Alignment:* Keep your knees in line with your toes to avoid strain.

- *Back Position:* Maintain a neutral spine and avoid rounding your back.

- *Depth:* Lower your body until your thighs are parallel to the ground but go as deep as your flexibility allows without compromising form.

Common Mistakes to Avoid

- *Knees Caving In*: Ensure your knees stay in line with your toes.

- *Heels Lifting:* Keep your heels flat on the ground throughout the movement.

- *Leaning Forward:* Keep your chest up and avoid leaning too far forward.

RUSSIAN TWISTS

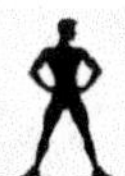  **How to Perform Standing Body Twists**

1. *Starting Position:* Stand with your feet shoulder-width apart. Keep your knees slightly bent. Place your hands on your hips or extend your arms out to the sides at shoulder height.
2. *Twist Your Torso:* Engage your core muscles. Twist your torso to the right, keeping your hips facing forward. Return to the centre and then twist to the left.
3. *Controlled Movements*: Perform the twists in a slow and controlled manner. Focus on using your oblique muscles to twist rather than swinging your arms or using momentum.

Breathing Technique*:* Inhale as you prepare to twist. Exhale as you twist your torso to one side. Inhale as you return to the centre. Exhale as you twist to the other side.

Tips for Proper Form

- *Core Engagement:* Keep your core muscles engaged throughout the exercise to protect your lower back.

- *Hip Position:* Ensure your hips remain facing forward and do not rotate with your torso.

- *Controlled Movements:* Avoid using momentum; focus on controlled, deliberate movements.

Common Mistakes to Avoid

- *Using Momentum:* Swinging your arms or using momentum can reduce the effectiveness of the exercise and increase the risk of injury.

- *Rotating Hips:* Allowing your hips to rotate can reduce the engagement of your oblique muscles.

- *Fast Movements:* Performing the twists too quickly can lead to poor form and potential strain.

JUMP SQUATS

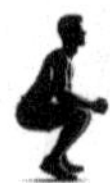

How to Perform Jump Squats

1. *Starting Position:* Stand with your feet shoulder-width apart. Keep your toes slightly pointed outwards. Place your hands behind your head or extend them in front of you for balance.
2. *Lower Your Body*: Engage your core and keep your chest up. Push your hips back and bend your knees to lower into a squat position. Ensure your thighs are parallel to the ground and your knees are tracking over your toes.
3. *Jump Up:* Explosively push through your heels to jump straight up. Extend your legs fully and reach maximum height. Swing your arms upward to help with the jump if they are not behind your head.
4. *Land Softly:* Land softly on the balls of your feet and immediately lower back into the squat position to absorb the impact. Ensure your knees are slightly bent upon landing to reduce stress on your joints.

Breathing Technique: Inhale as you lower your body into the squat. Exhale as you jump up. Inhale as you land and prepare for the next squat.

Tips for Proper Form

- *Knee Alignment:* Keep your knees in line with your toes to avoid strain.

- *Back Position:* Maintain a neutral spine and avoid rounding your back.

- *Controlled Movements:* Focus on controlled landings to protect your joints.

Common Mistakes to Avoid

- *Knees Caving In*: Ensure your knees stay in line with your toes during the squat and landing.

- *Heels Lifting:* Keep your heels flat on the ground during the squat phase.

- *Hard Landings:* Land softly to reduce the impact on your joints.

PUSH-UPS

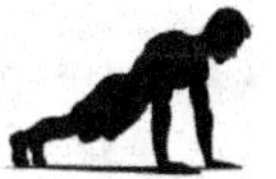

How to Perform Push-Ups

1. *Starting Position:* Begin in a plank position with your hands placed slightly wider than shoulder width apart. Keep your feet together or slightly apart for balance. Ensure your body forms a straight line from your head to your heels.
2. *Lower Your Body:* Engage your core and keep your back flat. Bend your elbows to lower your body towards the ground. Keep your elbows at a 45-degree angle to your body. Lower yourself until your chest nearly touches the ground.
3. *Push Back Up:* Push through your palms to straighten your arms and return to the starting position. Ensure your body remains in a straight line throughout the movement.
4. *Initially* bend your knees into a kneeling position, palms in the ground with arms in line with your shoulders or slightly out to create a square or a box position and attempt the push up

Breathing Technique: Inhale as you lower your body towards the ground. Exhale as you push back up to the starting position.

Tips for Proper Form

- *Hand Placement:* Keep your hands slightly wider than shoulder-width apart.

- *Body Alignment:* Maintain a straight line from your head to your heels.

- *Elbow Position:* Keep your elbows at a 45-degree angle to your body to reduce shoulder strain.

Common Mistakes to Avoid

- *Sagging Hips:* Keep your core engaged to prevent your hips from sagging.

- *Flared Elbows:* Avoid letting your elbows flare out too much, which can strain your shoulders.

- *Incomplete Range of Motion:* Lower your body until your chest nearly touches the ground for a full range of motion.

CALF RAISES

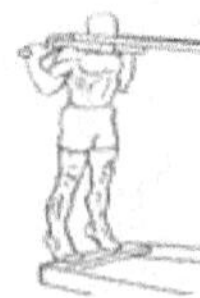

How to Perform Standing Calf Raises

1. *Starting Position:* Stand upright with your feet hip-width apart. Keep your hands on your hips or hold onto a stable surface for balance.
2. *Raise Your Heels*: Engage your core and keep your legs straight. Slowly raise your heels off the ground, lifting your body onto the balls of your feet. Hold the top position for a moment, feeling the contraction in your calf muscles.
3. *Lower Your Heels:* Slowly lower your heels back to the starting position. Ensure you lower your heels in a controlled manner to maintain balance.

Breathing Technique: Inhale as you lower your heels back to the ground. Exhale as you raise your heels.

Tips for Proper Form

- *Controlled Movements:* Perform the exercise slowly and with control to maximize muscle engagement.

- *Full Range of Motion:* Raise your heels as high as possible and lower them fully to stretch the calf muscles.

- *Balance:* Use a stable surface for support if needed to maintain balance.

Common Mistakes to Avoid

- *Bouncing:* Avoid bouncing up and down; focus on slow, controlled movements.

- *Leaning Forward:* Keep your body upright and avoid leaning forward.

- *Partial Range of Motion:* Ensure you go through the full range of motion for maximum benefit.

FULL PLANK

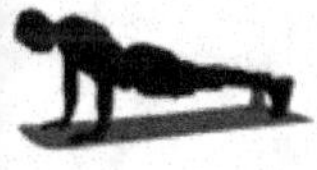

How to Perform a Full Plank

1. *Starting Position:* Begin on all fours with your hands directly under your shoulders and your knees under your hips. Step your feet back one at a time to extend your legs fully, coming into a high plank position. Your body should form a straight line from your head to your heels.
2. *Engage Your Core:* Tighten your abdominal muscles to keep your body straight. Avoid letting your hips sag or rise too high.
3. *Hold the Position:* Keep your neck in a neutral position by looking at a spot on the floor about a foot in front of your hands. Hold this position for the desired amount of time, maintaining a steady breath.

Breathing Technique: Inhale and exhale steadily throughout the hold. Focus on deep, controlled breaths to maintain stability.

Tips for Proper Form

- *Body Alignment:* Ensure your body forms a straight line from your head to your heels.

- *Shoulder Position:* Keep your shoulders directly above your wrists.

- *Core Engagement:* Maintain a tight core to prevent your hips from sagging.

Common Mistakes to Avoid

- *Sagging Hips:* Keep your hips in line with your body to avoid lower back strain.

- *Raised Hips:* Avoid lifting your hips too high, which reduces the effectiveness of the exercise.

- *Neck Position:* Keep your neck neutral and avoid looking up or down excessively

TRICEP DIPS

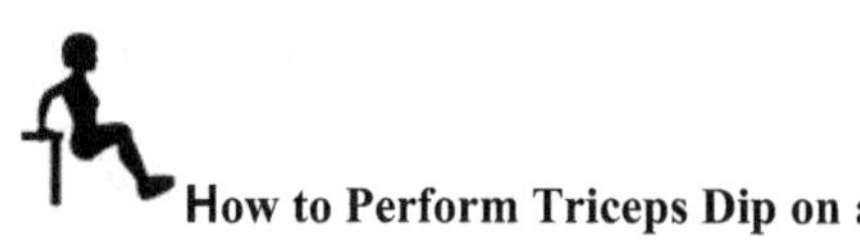 **How to Perform Triceps Dip on a Bench**

1. *Starting Position:* Sit on the edge of a bench with your hands placed next to your hips, fingers pointing forward. Extend your legs out in front of you with your heels on the ground. Slide your hips off the bench, supporting your weight with your hands.
2. *Lower Your Body:* Bend your elbows to lower your body towards the ground. Keep your elbows pointing straight back and your shoulders down. Lower yourself until your upper arms are parallel to the ground.
3. *Push Back Up:* Push through your palms to straighten your arms and lift your body back to the starting position. Keep your elbows slightly bent at the top to maintain tension on your triceps.

Breathing Technique: Inhale as you lower your body towards the ground. Exhale as you push back up to the starting position.

Tips for Proper Form

- *Elbow Position:* Keep your elbows pointing straight back to target the triceps effectively.

- *Shoulder Position:* Avoid shrugging your shoulders; keep them down and away from your ears.

- *Controlled Movements:* Perform the exercise in a slow and controlled manner to avoid strain.

Common Mistakes to Avoid

- *Elbows Flaring Out:* Ensure your elbows stay close to your body to focus on the triceps.

- *Partial Range of Motion:* Lower your body until your upper arms are parallel to the ground for full range of motion.

- *Shoulder Shrugging:* Keep your shoulders down to avoid unnecessary strain.

LUNGE SPLIT JUMPS

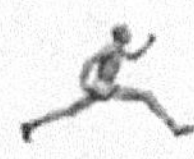

How to Perform Lunge Split Jumps

1. *Starting Position:* Stand upright with your feet together. Keep your hands on your hips or by your sides for balance.
2. *Lunge Position:* Step your right foot forward into a lunge position. Lower your body until your right thigh is parallel to the ground and your left knee is just above the floor.
3. *Jump and Switch:* Explosively jump up, switching your legs in mid-air. Land softly with your left foot forward in a lunge position and your right foot back. Ensure your knees are bent to absorb the impact.
4. *Repeat:* Continue jumping and switching legs for the desired number of repetitions. **Breathing**

Technique

- Inhale as you lower into the lunge. Exhale as you jump and switch legs.

Tips for Proper Form

Knee Alignment: Ensure your front knee does not extend past your toes.

- *Torso Position:* Keep your torso upright and avoid leaning forward.

- *Controlled Movements:* Focus on controlled landings to maintain balance and reduce the risk of injury.

Common Mistakes to Avoid

- *Knees Caving In:* Keep your knees in line with your toes to avoid strain.

- *Hard Landings:* Land softly to reduce the impact on your joints.

- *Leaning Forward:* Maintain an upright torso to protect your lower back.

SIDE LUNGES

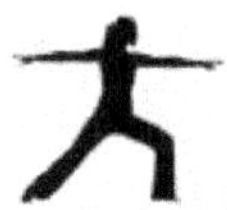

How to Perform Side Lunges

1. *Starting Position:* Stand upright with your feet hip-width apart. Keep your hands on your hips or clasp them in front of your chest for balance.
2. *Step to the Side:* Take a big step to the right with your right foot. Keep your left leg straight and your right knee bent as you lower your body.
3. *Lower Your Body:* Push your hips back and bend your right knee until your right thigh is parallel to the ground. Ensure your right knee is directly above your right ankle. Keep your left leg straight and your left foot flat on the ground.
4. *Return to Starting Position:* Push through your right heel to return to the starting position. Repeat the movement on the left side.

Breathing Technique: *Inhale as you step to the side and lower your body. Exhale as you push back up to the starting position.*

Tips for Proper Form

- *Knee Alignment:* Ensure your bent knee does not extend past your toes.

- *Torso Position:* Keep your torso upright and avoid leaning forward.

- *Controlled Movements:* Perform the exercise slowly and with control to maintain balance and engage the muscles effectively.

Common Mistakes to Avoid

- *Overstepping:* Taking too large a step can cause imbalance.

- *Knee Position:* Allowing the bent knee to go past the toes can lead to knee strain.

- *Leaning Forward:* This can put unnecessary stress on your lower back.

VERTICAL LEG CRUNCHES

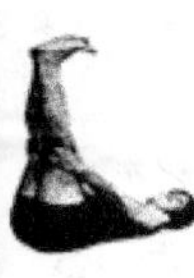 **How to Perform Vertical Leg Crunches**

1. *Starting Position:* Lie flat on your back on a mat. Extend your legs straight up towards the ceiling, keeping them together. Place your hands behind your head with your elbows pointing out to the sides.
2. *Engage Your Core:* Tighten your abdominal muscles to prepare for the movement.
3. *Lift Your Shoulders:* Lift your shoulders and upper back off the ground by contracting your abs. Keep your legs straight and pointed towards the ceiling. Avoid pulling on your neck with your hands; use your abs to lift.
4. *Lower Back Down:* Slowly lower your shoulders and upper back to the starting position. Keep your legs extended and your core engaged throughout the movement.

Breathing Technique: Inhale as you lower your shoulders back to the ground. Exhale as you lift your shoulders and upper back off the ground.

Tips for Proper Form

- *Neck Position:* Avoid pulling on your neck with your hands; keep your neck in a neutral position.

- *Leg Position:* Keep your legs straight and pointed towards the ceiling.

- *Controlled Movements:* Perform the exercise slowly and with control to maximize muscle engagement.

Common Mistakes to Avoid

- *Pulling on the Neck:* Use your abs to lift your shoulders, not your hands.

- *Fast Movements:* Perform the exercise slowly to maintain control and effectiveness.

- *Leg Movement:* Keep your legs stable and point towards the ceiling throughout the exercise.

SINGLE LEG LIFTS

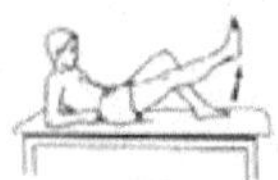

How to Perform Single Leg Lifts (Supine)

1. *Starting Position:* Lie flat on your back on a mat. Extend your legs straight out in front of you. Place your arms by your sides with your palms facing down for support.
2. *Engage Your Core:* Tighten your abdominal muscles to stabilize your lower back.
3. *Lift One Leg:* Keeping your left leg straight on the mat, slowly lift your right leg towards the ceiling. Raise your right leg until it forms a 90-degree angle with your body or as high as your flexibility allows. Ensure your lower back remains in contact with the mat.
4. *Lower Your Leg:* Slowly lower your right leg back to the starting position without letting it touch the ground. Repeat the movement with your left leg.

Breathing Technique: Inhale as you lower your leg back to the mat. Exhale as you lift your leg towards the ceiling.

Tips for Proper Form

- *Core Engagement:* Keep your core muscles engaged throughout the exercise to protect your lower back.

- *Leg Control:* Move your leg in a slow and controlled manner to maximize muscle engagement.

- *Lower Back Position:* Ensure your lower back stays in contact with the mat to avoid strain.

Common Mistakes to Avoid

- Arching the Back: Keep your lower back pressed into the mat to prevent strain.

- Fast Movements: Perform the exercise slowly to maintain control and effectiveness.

- Partial Range of Motion: Lift your leg as high as your flexibility allows without compromising form.

ABDOMEN SIT-UPS

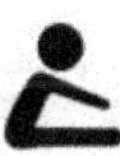

How to Perform Ab Sit-Ups

1. *Starting Position:* Lie flat on your back on a mat. Bend your knees and place your feet flat on the ground, hip-width apart. Cross your arms over your chest or place your hands behind your head without pulling on your neck.
2. *Engage Your Core:* Tighten your abdominal muscles to prepare for the movement.
3. *Lift Your Upper Body:* Using your abs, lift your upper body off the ground towards your knees. Keep your feet flat on the ground and avoid using momentum. Lift until your chest is close to your thighs.
4. *Lower Back Down:* Slowly lower your upper body back to the starting position. Ensure your lower back touches the mat before your shoulders.

Breathing Technique: Inhale as you lower your upper body back to the mat. Exhale as you lift your upper body towards your knees.

Tips for Proper Form

- *Neck Position:* Avoid pulling on your neck with your hands; keep your neck in a neutral position.

- *Core Engagement:* Focus on using your abdominal muscles to lift your body, not your arms or momentum.

- *Controlled Movements:* Perform the exercise slowly and with control to maximize muscle engagement.

Common Mistakes to Avoid

- *Pulling on the Neck:* Use your abs to lift your upper body, not your hands.

- *Using Momentum:* Avoid swinging your body; focus on controlled movements.

- *Partial Range of Motion:* Lift your upper body fully to engage your abs effectively.

BICYCLE CRUNCHES

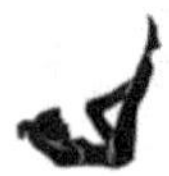

How to Perform Bicycle Crunches

1. *Starting Position:* Lie flat on your back on a mat. Place your hands behind your head, elbows pointing out to the sides. Lift your legs off the ground, bending your knees at a 90-degree angle.
2. *Engage Your Core:* Tighten your abdominal muscles to stabilize your lower back.
3. *Begin the Movement:* Bring your right elbow towards your left knee while simultaneously straightening your right leg. Twist your torso to bring your elbow and knee together, engaging your oblique muscles.
4. *Switch Sides:* Return to the starting position and then bring your left elbow towards your right knee while straightening your left leg. Continue alternating sides in a smooth, controlled motion.

Breathing Technique: *Inhale as you return to the starting position. Exhale as you twist and bring your elbow to your knee.*

Tips for Proper Form

- *Controlled Movements:* Perform the exercise slowly and with control to maximize muscle engagement.

- *Elbow Position:* Keep your elbows wide and avoid pulling on your neck.

- *Leg Movement:* Fully extend your leg with each repetition to engage your lower abs

Common Mistakes to Avoid

- *Pulling on the Neck:* Use your abs to twist your torso, not your hands.

- *Fast Movements:* Avoid rushing through the exercise; focus on controlled, deliberate movements.

- *Partial Range of Motion:* Ensure you twist fully to engage your oblique muscles effectively.

WALL PUSH-UPS

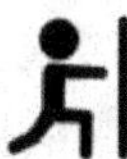

How to Perform Wall Push-Ups

1. *Starting Position:* Stand facing a wall at arm's length distance. Place your hands on the wall at shoulder height and shoulder width apart. Keep your feet together or slightly apart for balance.
2. *Engage Your Core:* Tighten your abdominal muscles to maintain a straight line from your head to your heels.
3. *Lower Your Body:* Bend your elbows and lean your body towards the wall. Keep your elbows at a 45-degree angle to your body. Lower yourself until your nose is close to the wall.
4. *Push Back Up:* Push through your palms to straighten your arms and return to the starting position. Ensure your body remains in a straight line throughout the movement.

Breathing Technique: Inhale as you lower your body towards the wall. Exhale as you push back up to the starting position.

Tips for Proper Form

- *Hand Placement:* Keep your hands at shoulder height and shoulder-width apart.

- *Body Alignment:* Maintain a straight line from your head to your heels.

- *Elbow Position:* Keep your elbows at a 45-degree angle to your body to reduce shoulder strain.

Common Mistakes to Avoid

- *Sagging Hips:* Keep your core engaged to prevent your hips from sagging.

- *Flared Elbows:* Avoid letting your elbows flare out too much, which can strain your shoulders.

- *Incomplete Range of Motion:* Lower your body until your nose is close to the wall for a full range of motion.

INCLINE PUSH-UPS

How to Perform Incline Push-Ups

1. *Starting Position:* Find a sturdy surface like a bench, step, or low wall. Place your hands on the edge of the surface, slightly wider than shoulder-width apart. Walk your feet back until your body forms a straight line from your head to your heels. Keep your arms straight and your core engaged.
2. *Lower Your Body:* Bend your elbows to lower your chest towards the edge of the surface. Keep your elbows at a 45-degree angle to your body. Lower yourself until your chest nearly touches the surface.
3. *Push Back Up:* Push through your palms to straighten your arms and return to the starting position. Ensure your body remains in a straight line throughout the movement.

Breathing Technique: Inhale as you lower your body towards the surface. Exhale as you push back up to the starting position.

Tips for Proper Form

- *Hand Placement:* Keep your hands slightly wider than shoulder-width apart.

- *Body Alignment:* Maintain a straight line from your head to your heels.

- *Elbow Position:* Keep your elbows at a 45-degree angle to your body to reduce shoulder strain.

Common Mistakes to Avoid

- *Sagging Hips:* Keep your core engaged to prevent your hips from sagging.

- *Flared Elbows:* Avoid letting your elbows flare out too much, which can strain your shoulders.

- *Incomplete Range of Motion:* Lower your body until your chest nearly touches the surface for full range of motion.

ABDOMEN CRUNCHES WITH LEG AT 90% ANGLE

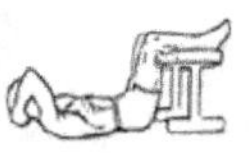 **How to Perform Ab Crunches with Knees at Right Angle**

1. *Starting Position:* Lie flat on your back on a mat. Bend your knees and lift your legs so that your thighs are perpendicular to the ground and your shins are parallel to the ground, forming a 90degree angle. Place your hands behind your head with your elbows pointing out to the sides.
2. *Engage Your Core:* Tighten your abdominal muscles to prepare for the movement.
3. *Lift Your Shoulders:* Using your abs, lift your shoulders and upper back off the ground. Keep your lower back pressed into the mat. Avoid pulling on your neck with your hands; use your abs to lift.
4. *Lower Back Down:* Slowly lower your shoulders and upper back to the starting position. Keep your legs in the 90-degree position throughout the exercise.

Breathing Technique: Inhale as you lower your shoulders back to the mat. Exhale as you lift your shoulders and upper back off the ground.

Tips for Proper Form

- *Neck Position:* Avoid pulling on your neck with your hands; keep your neck in a neutral position.

- *Core Engagement:* Focus on using your abdominal muscles to lift your body, not your arms or momentum.

- Leg Position: Keep your legs stable and at a 90-degree angle throughout the exercise.

Common Mistakes to Avoid

- *Pulling on the Neck:* Use your abs to lift your shoulders, not your hands.

- *Using Momentum:* Avoid swinging your body; focus on controlled movements.

- *Leg Movement:* Keep your legs stable and avoid letting them move during the exercise.

BIRD DOG EXERCISE

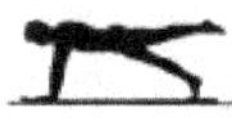 **Bird Dog Exercise for Beginners**

1. *Starting Position:* Begin on all fours with your hands directly under your shoulders and your knees under your hips. Keep your back flat and your core engaged.
2. *Extend Opposite Arm and Leg:* Slowly extend your right arm forward and your left leg backward, keeping them in line with your body. Ensure your hips remain level and your back stays flat.
3. *Hold and Return:* Hold the position for a few seconds, focusing on balance and stability. Slowly return to the starting position and repeat with your left arm and right leg.

Breathing Technique: Inhale as you extend your arm and leg. Exhale as you return to the starting position.

Tips for Proper Form

- *Core Engagement:* Keep your core muscles engaged to maintain stability.

- *Hip Position:* Ensure your hips stay level and do not rotate.

- *Controlled Movements:* Perform the exercise slowly to focus on balance and control.   **Common Mistakes to Avoid**

- *Arching the Back:* Keep your back flat to avoid strain.

- *Rotating Hips:* Maintain level hips to engage your core effectively.

- *Fast Movements:* Perform the exercise slowly to maintain control and balance.

Bird Dog Exercise Advanced *Starting Position:* Begin on all fours with your hands directly under your shoulders and your knees under your hips. Keep your back flat and your core engaged. *Extend Opposite Arm and Leg with Resistance:* Attach a resistance band to your right hand and left foot. Slowly extend your right arm forward and your left leg backward against the resistance, keeping them in line with your body. Ensure your hips remain level and your back stays flat. *Hold and Return:* Hold the position for a few seconds, focusing on balance and stability. Slowly return to the starting position and repeat with your left arm and right leg.

OBLIQUE CRUNCHES

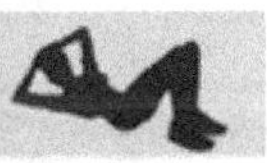 **How to Perform Oblique Crunches**

1. *Starting Position:* Lie flat on your back on a mat. Bend your knees and place your feet flat on the ground, hip-width apart. Place your hands behind your head with your elbows pointing out to the sides.
2. *Engage Your Core:* Tighten your abdominal muscles to prepare for the movement.
3. *Lift and Twist:* Lift your shoulders and upper back off the ground while twisting your torso to bring your right elbow towards your left knee. Keep your left leg bent and your right leg extended.
4. *Return to Starting Position:* Lower your shoulders and upper back to the starting position. Repeat the movement on the opposite side, bringing your left elbow towards your right knee.

Breathing Technique: Inhale as you lower your shoulders back to the mat. Exhale as you lift and twist your torso.

Tips for Proper Form

- *Neck Position:* Avoid pulling on your neck with your hands; keep your neck in a neutral position.

- *Core Engagement:* Focus on using your oblique muscles to twist your torso, not your arms or momentum.

- *Controlled Movements:* Perform the exercise slowly and with control to maximize muscle engagement.

Common Mistakes to Avoid

- *Pulling on the Neck:* Use your abs to lift and twist your torso, not your hands.

- *Using Momentum:* Avoid swinging your body; focus on controlled movements.

- *Partial Range of Motion:* Twist fully to engage your oblique muscles effectively.

SIDE PLANK

How to Perform a Side Plank

1. *Starting Position:* Lie on your side with your legs extended and stacked on top of each other. Place your elbow directly under your shoulder, with your forearm perpendicular to your body. Your other hand can rest on your hip or extend towards the ceiling for added balance.
2. *Lift Your Hips:* Engage your core and lift your hips off the ground, forming a straight line from your head to your feet. Ensure your body remains in a straight line without sagging or bending.
3. *Hold the Position:* Hold this position for the desired amount of time, maintaining a steady breath. Keep your core tight and your hips lifted.
4. *Switch Sides:* Lower your hips back to the ground and switch to the other side to repeat the exercise.

Breathing Technique: Inhale and exhale steadily throughout the hold. Focus on deep, controlled breaths to maintain stability.

Tips for Proper Form

- *Body Alignment:* Ensure your body forms a straight line from your head to your feet.

- *Shoulder Position:* Keep your shoulder directly above your elbow to avoid strain.

- *Core Engagement:* Maintain a tight core to keep your hips lifted and stable.

Common Mistakes to Avoid

- *Sagging Hips*: Keep your hips in line with your body to avoid lower back strain.

- *Rotating Shoulders:* Ensure your shoulders stay stacked and do not rotate forward or backward.

- *Neck Position:* Keep your neck neutral and avoid looking up or down excessively.

HIGH KNEE

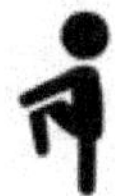

How to Perform High Knees

1. *Starting Position:* Stand upright with your feet hip-width apart. Keep your arms at your sides or bent at a 90-degree angle.
2. *Lift Your Knees:* Quickly lift your right knee towards your chest. As you lower your right knee, lift your left knee towards your chest. Continue alternating knees in a running motion.
3. *Arm Movement:* Swing your arms in sync with your legs, as if you are running. Keep your elbows bent at a 90-degree angle.

Breathing Technique: Inhale and exhale steadily throughout the exercise. Focus on deep, controlled breaths to maintain rhythm and endurance.

Tips for Proper Form

- *Core Engagement:* Keep your core muscles engaged to maintain balance and stability.

- *Knee Height:* Lift your knees as high as possible, ideally to hip level.

- *Controlled Movements:* Perform the exercise quickly but with control to avoid injury.

Common Mistakes to Avoid

- *Leaning Back:* Keep your torso upright and avoid leaning back.

- *Low Knees:* Ensure you lift your knees high enough to engage your core and leg muscles effectively.

- *Flat Feet:* Land on the balls of your feet to reduce impact on your joints.

BUTT KICKS

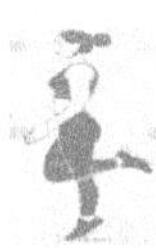

How to Perform Butt Kicks

1. *Starting Position:* Stand upright with your feet hip-width apart. Keep your arms at your sides or bent at a 90-degree angle.
2. *Kick Your Heels:* Quickly lift your right heel towards your glutes. As you lower your right heel, lift your left heel towards your glutes. Continue alternating heels in a running motion.
3. *Arm Movement:* Swing your arms in sync with your legs, as if you are running. Keep your elbows bent at a 90-degree angle.

Breathing Technique: Inhale and exhale steadily throughout the exercise. Focus on deep, controlled breaths to maintain rhythm and endurance.

Tips for Proper Form

- *Core Engagement:* Keep your core muscles engaged to maintain balance and stability.

- *Heel Height:* Lift your heels as high as possible towards your glutes.

- *Controlled Movements:* Perform the exercise quickly but with control to avoid injury.

Common Mistakes to Avoid

- *Leaning Forward:* Keep your torso upright and avoid leaning forward.

- *Low Heels:* Ensure you lift your heels high enough to engage your hamstrings effectively.

- *Flat Feet:* Land on the balls of your feet to reduce impact on your joints.

JACK KNIFE sit-ups

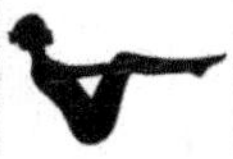

How to Perform Jackknife Sit-Ups

1. *Starting Position:* Lie flat on your back on a mat. Extend your arms straight back behind your head. Extend your legs straight out in front of you.
2. *Engage Your Core:* Tighten your abdominal muscles to prepare for the movement.
3. *Lift Your Upper Body and Legs:* Simultaneously lift your upper body and legs towards each other. Aim to touch your hands to your feet at the top of the movement. Keep your legs straight and your arms extended.
4. *Lower Back Down:* Slowly lower your upper body and legs back to the starting position. Ensure your lower back touches the mat before your shoulders.

Breathing Technique Inhale as you lower your upper body and legs back to the mat. Exhale as you lift your upper body and legs towards each other.

Tips for Proper Form

- *Core Engagement:* Focus on using your abdominal muscles to lift your body, not your arms or momentum.

- *Leg and Arm Position:* Keep your legs and arms straight throughout the movement.

- *Controlled Movements:* Perform the exercise slowly and with control to maximize muscle engagement.

Common Mistakes to Avoid

- *Using Momentum:* Avoid swinging your body; focus on controlled movements.

- *Bending Knees:* Keep your legs straight to engage your core effectively.

- *Partial Range of Motion:* Lift your upper body and legs fully to engage your abs effectively.

DOWNWARD FACING DOG EXERCISE

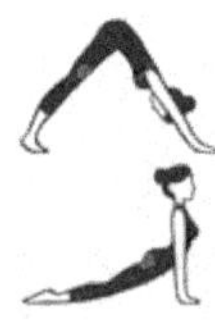

How to Perform Downward Facing Dog

1. *Starting Position*: Begin on all fours with your hands directly under your shoulders and your knees under your hips. Spread your fingers wide and press firmly into the mat.
2. *Lift Your Hips:* Tuck your toes under and lift your hips towards the ceiling. Straighten your legs as much as possible, forming an inverted V-shape with your body.
3. *Align Your Body:* Keep your head between your upper arms, ears aligned with your upper arms. Press your heels towards the ground, even if they don't touch. Engage your core and keep your spine long.
4. *Hold the Position:* Hold this position for several breaths, maintaining a steady and deep breathing pattern. Focus on lengthening your spine and pressing your chest towards your thighs.

Breathing Technique: Inhale deeply through your nose as you lift your hips and lengthen your spine. Exhale through your nose as you press your heels towards the ground and deepen the stretch.

Tips for Proper Form

- *Hand Placement:* Spread your fingers wide and press evenly through your palms.

- *Shoulder Position:* Keep your shoulders away from your ears and your neck relaxed.

- *Leg Position:* Keep your legs straight but avoid locking your knees.

Common Mistakes to Avoid

- *Rounded Back:* Focus on lengthening your spine rather than rounding your back.

- *Tension in Shoulders:* Keep your shoulders relaxed and away from your ears.

- *Heels Lifting:* It's okay if your heels don't touch the ground, but aim to press them down gently.

PRONE BACK EXTENSION

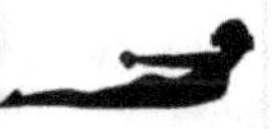 **How to Perform the Prone Back Extension**

1. *Starting Position*: Lie face down on a mat with your legs extended and the tops of your feet flat on the ground. Place your hands under your shoulders with your elbows close to your body.
2. *Engage Your Core:* Tighten your abdominal muscles to support your lower back.
3. *Lift Your Upper Torso:* Press through your hands to lift your chest off the ground. Keep your elbows slightly bent and your shoulders relaxed. Lift only as high as is comfortable, ensuring your lower body remains firmly on the mat.
4. *Hold the Position:* Hold the stretch for a few breaths, focusing on lengthening your spine and opening your chest. Keep your gaze forward or slightly upward, avoiding any strain on your neck.
5. *Lower Back Down:* Slowly lower your upper body back to the starting position. Repeat the movement for the desired number of repetitions.

Breathing Technique: Inhale as you lift your upper torso off the ground. Exhale as you lower your upper torso back to the mat.

Tips for Proper Form

- *Hand Placement:* Keep your hands under your shoulders and your elbows close to your body.

- *Core Engagement:* Engage your core muscles to protect your lower back.

- *Controlled Movements:* Perform the exercise slowly and with control to maximize the stretch.

Common Mistakes to Avoid

- *Overarching the Back:* Lift only as high as is comfortable to avoid straining your lower back.

- *Tension in Shoulders*: Keep your shoulders relaxed and away from your ears.

- *Fast Movements:* Perform the exercise slowly to maintain control and effectiveness

CHAPTER 4

WARM UP AND GET SET

You've now reached the exciting point where you're ready to start exercising! If you're generally healthy with no specific health issues, you can jump right into the following program. However, if you have any conditions like back pain, knee pain, diabetes, or high blood pressure, it's best to start with the stretching segment for a few weeks before moving on to the Daily Workout Program.

Warm-Up. Warming up is crucial as it gradually increases your heart rate, balances blood flow throughout your body, improves flexibility, and prepares you for more intense movements. It also helps prevent injuries and ensures you burn the maximum number of calories during your workout. If you prefer not to do slow, part-bypart warm-up movements, **5 to 10 minutes** of jogging or walking on a treadmill or elliptical can also get your body ready for a vigorous workout, especially if you're already fit.

Special Instructions: Keep a bottle of cool water handy and take a sip whenever your throat feels dry.
If during the workout you feel your heart rate is too high, you can't speak freely, or you feel lightheaded, it's a sign to slow down. If the discomfort continues, stop exercising or switch to an easier exercise.

If this is your first time exercising, you might need a day's rest after 2-3 days during the first week as your body gets accustomed to the new routine. However, if you're feeling good and don't have any body aches, continue with your routine and take a day's break at least once a week.

Attire: Wear breathable and comfortable clothes. For exercises involving jumps, fast running, or those that place stress on the lower body, a good pair of shoes and socks are recommended. For the stretching segment, bare feet are more comfortable. Use a mat for floor exercises.

SAMPLE WARM-UP EXERCISES

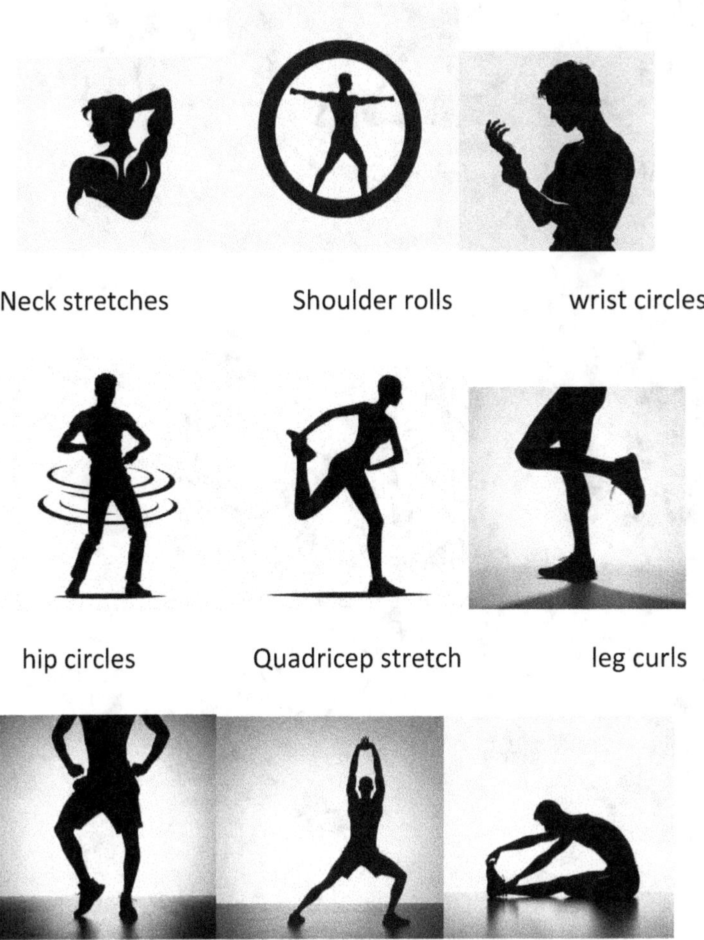

Neck stretches	Shoulder rolls	wrist circles
hip circles	Quadricep stretch	leg curls

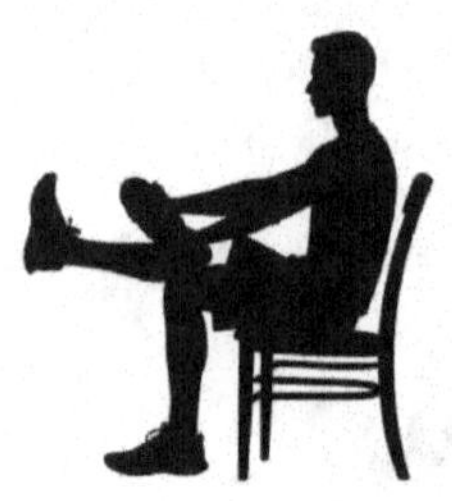

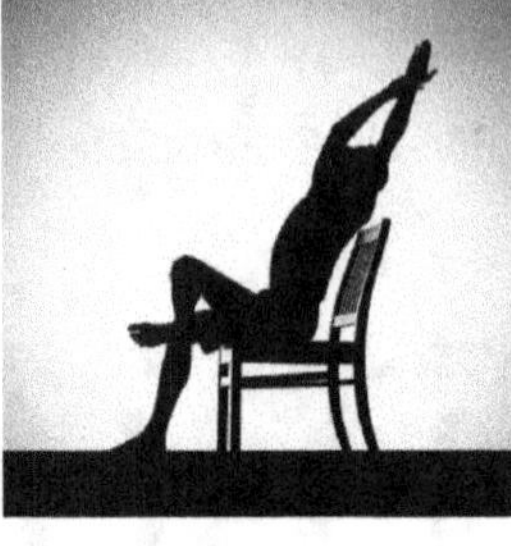

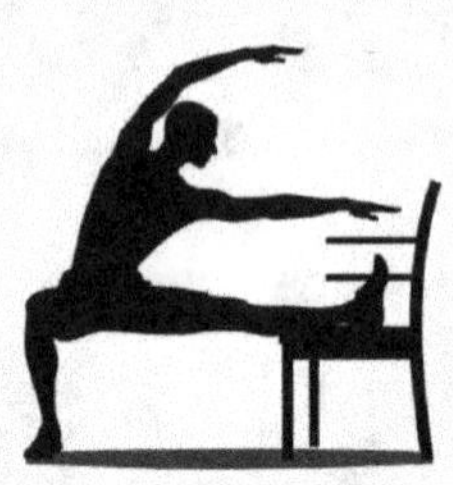

Ankle circles   side lunges   hamstring stretch

SEATED CHAIR MOVEMENTS

GLUTES AND KNEES   UPPER BODY   HAMSTRING AND SIDE

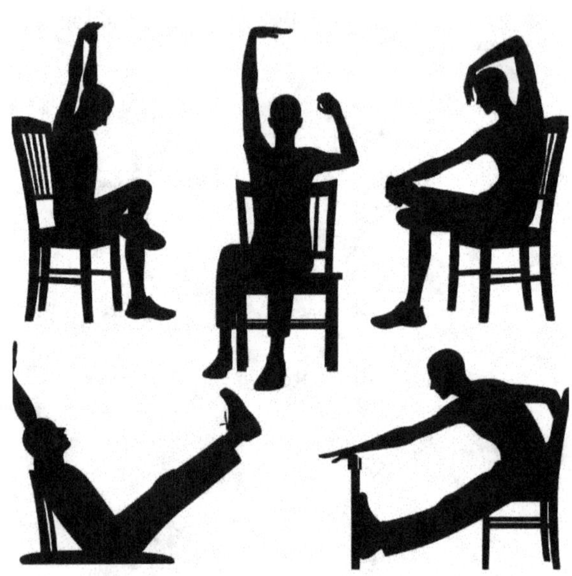

SIMPLE MOVEMENTS AS PER YOUR COMFORT AND FITNESS LEVEL

CHAPTER 5

20 MINUTE WORKOUTs

DAY 1 QUICK REFERENCE WORKOUT TABLE

	WARM-UP	
	JUMPING JACKS 50	LUNGES(EACH LEG)-20
	SQUATS 15	RUSSIAN TWIST-70
	JUMP SQUATS - 5	PUSH-UPS 25
	STANDING CALF RAISES-20	PLANK -30 SECS
	TRICEP DIPS-20	LUNGE SPLIT JUMPS -10

Stretches for 5 to 10 minutes	

DAY 2 QUICK REFERENCE WORKOUT TABLE

WARM-UP	
JUMPING JACKS 60	SIDE LUNGES (EACH LEG-15)
VERTICAL LEG CRUNCHES-50	LEG LIFTS (EACH LEG)-15
SIT-UPS	BICYCLE CRUNCHES-50
TRICEP DIPS-15	WALL PUSH-UPS -25
SQUATS-20	RUSSIAN TWISTS-40

Stretches for 5 to 10 minutes	

DAY 3 QUICK REFERENCE WORKOUT TABLE

	WARM-UP	
	JUMPING JACKS – 90	SQUATS-30
	TRICEP DIPS – 20	INCLINE PUSH-UPS 25
	SIT-UPS 10	CRUNCHES-40
	BIRD DOG-30	OBLIQUE CRUNCHES-(each side10)

	PLANK -30 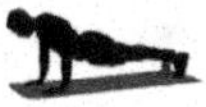	STANDING CALF RAISES-20 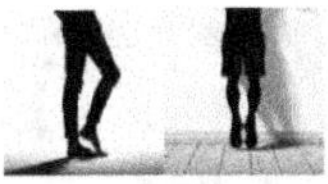
	Stretches for 5 to 10 minutes	

DAY 4 QUICK REFERENCE WORKOUT TABLE

	WARM-UP	
	JUMPING JACKS – 100 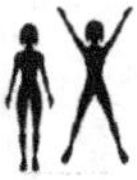	RUSSIAN TWIST-50 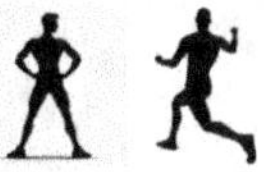
	VERTICAL LEG CRUNCHES -25 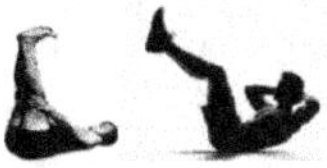	SIDE PLANK (EACH SIDE-15 SECS) 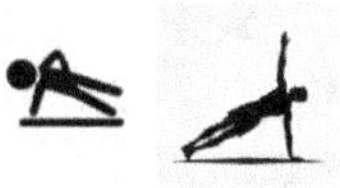
	CRUNCHES-30 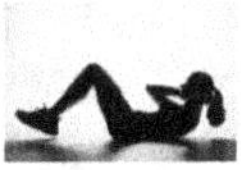	LUNGES SPLIT JUMP -10 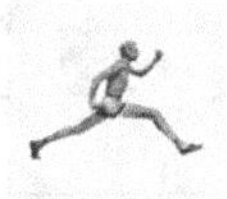
	SQUATS-20 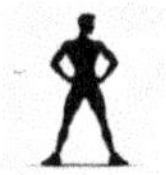	JUMP SQUATS-5 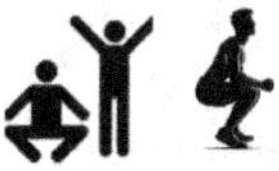

WALL PUSH-UPS-25	HIGH KNEE-40
Stretches for 5 to 10 minutes	

DAY 5 QUICK REFERENCE WORKOUT TABLE

WARM-UP	
JUMPING JACKS – 60	OBLIQUE CRUNCHES (EACH SIDE)20
SIT UPS -10	BUTT KICKS-30
TRICEP DIPS-10	JUMP SQUATS-5
SIDE LUNGES(EACH SIDE)20	JACK KNIFE SIT-UPS-15NOS

INCLINE PUSH-UPS 25 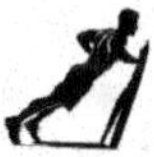	BICYCLE CRUNCHES-50 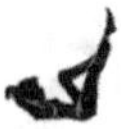
Stretches for 5 to 10 minutes	

DAY 6 QUICK REFERENCE WORKOUT TABLE

WARM-UP	
JUMPING JACKS – 50 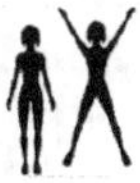	LUNGES EACH LEG -10 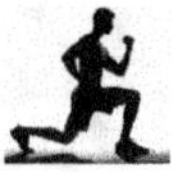
SQUATS-20 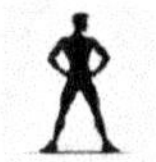	SIDE LUNGES (EACH SIDE-10) 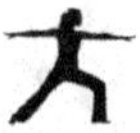
RUSSIAN TWIST-100 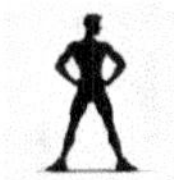 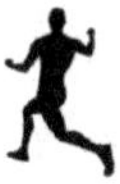	BIRD DOGS-20 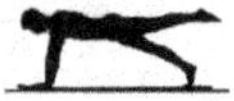
DOWNWARD FACING DOG-1 MIN 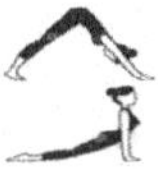	SIDE PLANK-15SEC 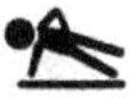 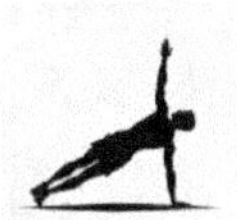

	JACK KNIFE SIT-UPS -15	INNER THIGH LIFTS(Each leg)–20
	Stretches for 5 to 10 minutes	

DAY 7 QUICK REFERENCE WORKOUT TABLE

	WARM-UP	
	JUMPING JACKS – 45	STANDING CALF RAISES-30SECS
	SQUATS-15	PUSHUPS 25
	JUMP SQUATS-5	BACKSTRETCH-30SEC
	RUSSIAN TWISTS-50	LUNGES EACH LEG10

PLANK-30 SEC	CRUNCHES-40
Stretches for 5 to 10 minutes	

CHAPTER 6

STRETCHES AND RELAXATION TECHNIQUES

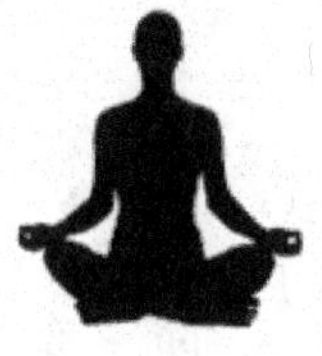

Various stretches and holds with health and fitness benefits

Stretches can be done before, during or after your workout. Stretches should be done in slow flow-like movements with continuous calm breathing. Do not overstrain or force the body to hold a pose. No sudden movements. Increase your range of movement once your body is familiar and able to hold a particular stretch. As you progress, hold each stretch initially for 30 seconds and then increase it to one or two minutes. You may need the support of the wall initially for certain exercises.

1. Slow Neck Stretches

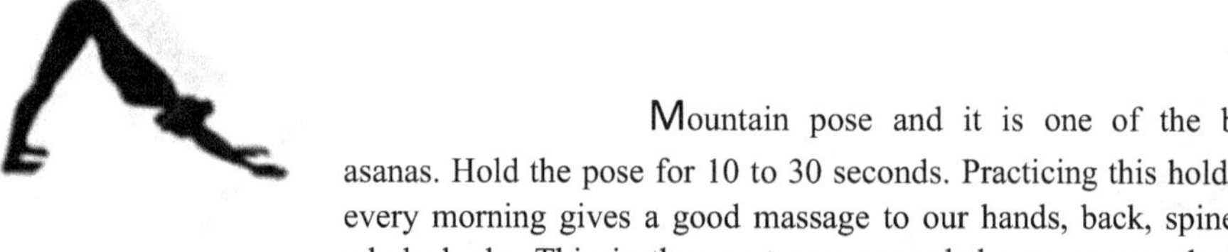

To start with one should get started with the basic exercises first like slow neck stretches. It is recommended to perform a few repetitions of slow neck movements side to side, ear to shoulder, slow circles, and reverse as it eases neck tension and strain. You can hold the pose for 10 seconds and can be easily done standing anywhere, even sitting on your chair!

2. Mountain Pose:

Mountain pose and it is one of the best yoga asanas. Hold the pose for 10 to 30 seconds. Practicing this hold regularly every morning gives a good massage to our hands, back, spine, and the whole body. This is the most recommended way to stretch the whole upper body and increase height in children as well.

3. Standing Forward Fold Pose :

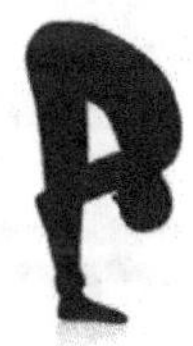

A forward-bending pose relaxes us from stress and anxiety. With the arm bound, this standing forward bend variation provides a deep shoulder stretch. Binding the hands also allows the arms to stretch and tighten the shoulders to relax. It also brings some blood back to the brain while giving a great stretch to the legs.

. 4. Triangle Pose:

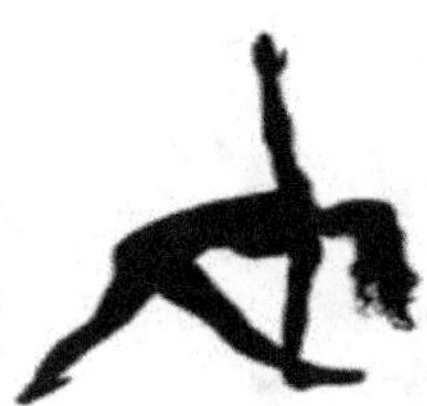

This stretches and strengthens the muscles along with improving the functions of our body. This is a good exercise even for pregnant women. It helps in reducing blood pressure, stress, and anxiety and improves the functions of the blood throughout the entire body. This improves our balance & concentration power. It also removes fat from the waist and thighs.

5.   Abdominal breathing:

The most recommended breathing exercise which cures our stomach disorder completely and we lose weight. Practicing for 5 minutes. Exhale fully while pulling your navel into your spine (as if you want your navel to touch your spine) hold for 3 seconds and inhale normally. Doing this regularly removes the toxins and increases metabolism. It also cures constipation, acidity, diabetes, Asthma, and all kinds of Respiratory troubles, sinus, and even hair loss. It is very effective in weight loss (mainly belly fat). This is a superb exercise for everyone.

6. Bound Angle Pose:

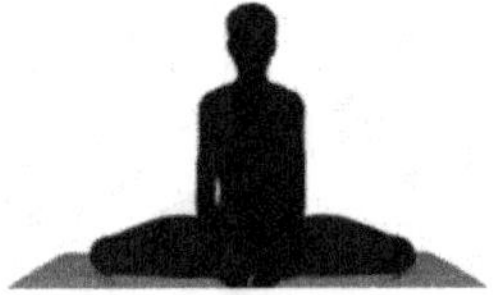

This pose for beginners helps to open up the hips and ease sciatica discomfort that can be made worse by sitting for long periods. The sciatic nerve starts in the lower back and runs down both legs, and sciatic nerve pain can occur when the nerve is somehow compressed. Long commutes and sitting for long periods exacerbate it.

***If you like what you have read up to now, kindly leave a good review.**

7. Forward Bend Pose:

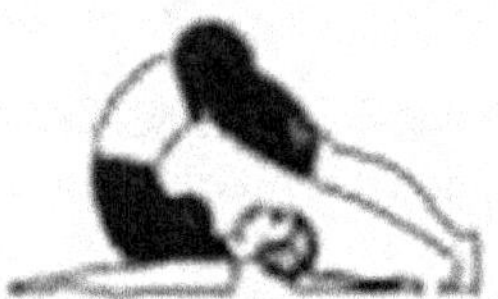

This exercise covers the stretching of the whole body from head to heels. It is recommended especially for women after delivery to reduce belly fat and toning the abdominal pelvic organs. It strengthens the back muscles as well as being very useful for increasing height. It stretches the spine and brings more flexibility to our body.

8. Plough Pose:

The Plough pose strengthens our back muscles and gives flexibility. It cures indigestion and constipation as well as reduces stress. It stimulates the abdominal organs and cures abdominal problems. People suffering from diabetes should do this regularly. It helps to make the spinal cord strong and flexible, strengthens the abdominal muscles, reduces stress, and cures the symptoms of menopause.

9. Half Plough Pose:

Half Plough Pose is done by lifting each leg and holding it for a few seconds.

It is good for improving the functions of abdominal organs. It stimulates abdominal organs very fast and cures constipation and indigestion. It also reduces belly fat and tones the thigh and hip muscles and overall abdominal muscles. It cures stomach disorders, improves digestion and appetite, removes gasses, and is useful to cure arthritis and lumbar spondylitis.

10. Cobra Pose:

Cobra pose gives an excellent result for those who want to lose weight and increase their metabolism. This pose improves the function of the liver, kidney, pancreas, and gallbladder. It cures insomnia (sleeping disorder), spine problems, indigestion, and constipation naturally. Those suffering from liver disease, headache, and poor blood circulation can be cured with this asana.

11.   The Raised-Leg hold:

The raised leg pose is beneficial for those having back pain and stomach disorders. You can initially put both your palms under your glutes to support your back while lifting your legs. It is good for strengthening the abdominal muscles. We can practice this hold by raising one leg at a time. For getting flat and strong abs this works as a wonder. It is helpful for those who suffer from gas problems, arthritis pain, heart problems, and waist & back pain.

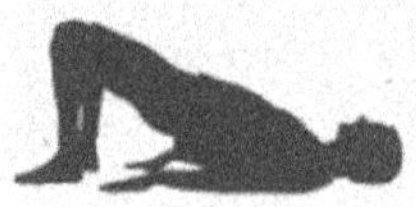

12.   Bridge hold:

We generally forget about doing any exercise meant for strengthening our legs as we care more about our upper body appearance. But we spend most of our hours on our legs only, so we should start a workout meant to strengthen our legs. This pose strengthens the legs, back neck, and chest. It provides great balancing power to our bodies. Keep breathing smoothly, inhale for 3 seconds if possible, and exhale for 5 seconds. Squeeze the glutes during the hold.

13. Child's Pose hold:

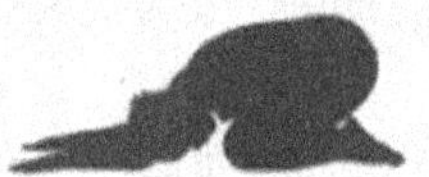

This stretch hold is a very simple yet calming pose which we can do in bed too. It is an excellent yoga exercise for those suffering from back pain as it stretches and relaxes the spine. It also stretches and strengthens the muscles of the hips, thighs, and ankles. Pregnant women and those suffering from high blood pressure should avoid doing it.

14. Warrior Pose hold:

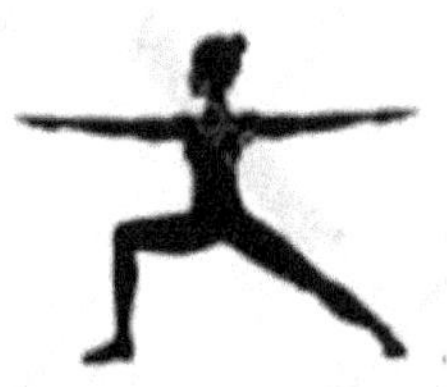

This pose looks like a soldier in the position of war. It is an excellent exercise for pregnant women. It gives flexibility to the entire body strengthens the legs, arms, and lower back, and tones the lower body. It also helps in increasing the stamina, concentration power, and balance of our body. It relieves us from the pain during the menstrual period.

15. Camel Pose stretch:

While performing this hold our body looks like the shape of a camel. It is especially good for back problems, relaxing the mind, blood circulation, respiratory system, endocrine, and nervous system. Initially just try to touch a single arm to the same leg at the back and change the hand and leg. Once your body is more flexible you can gently bend backward to hold both your feet while trusting your hip upwards.

It helps to increase chest size and lung capacity and brings flexibility to the chest, abdomen, and neck. It is beneficial for asthma patients and helps in reducing fats from the stomach.

16.   Boat Pose :

This asana is also called a Boat pose. It helps to strengthen the lungs, liver, and pancreas. It also helps to increase the circulation of blood and maintain the sugar level. It strengthens the muscles of the thigh, hips, neck, and shoulder and helps in reducing belly fat. It also improves the function of the kidney, thyroids, and prostate glands.

17. Cat Pose:

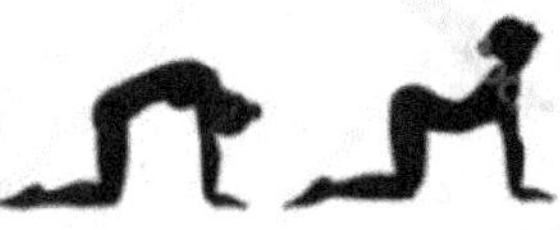

This cat pose is an excellent stretch in a yoga workout. It produces flexibility in our spine and releases us from back pain. It improves our blood circulation and digestion power. It is one of the best postures and tones our abdomen and helps in relaxing our mind.

18.   Tree Pose:

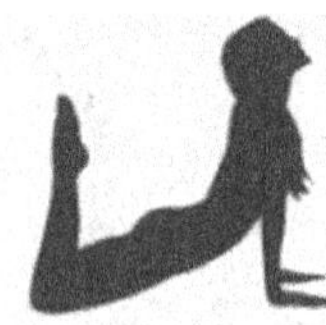

This posture helps to increase focus and concentration. For this, you need to stand on one foot while the other is locked behind the knees and your hands are raised above your head in a prayer pose. Initially let the toes of the bent knee touch the floor and as you get your balance gently lift your foot up. You can also hold your ear with a hand and only raise one hand and when you are well versed with this posture then raise both your hands over your head and join them in a prayer pose.

19.   Static tiger stretch:

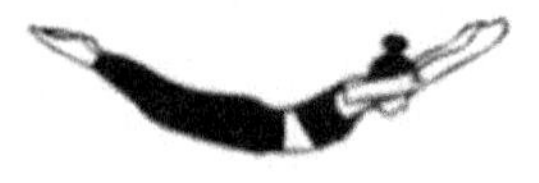

This is one good stretch to cure back pain issues. This especially focuses on the lower back area and stretches muscles and tissues over there causing a relief for pain in the area. Here you will first have to take the position of a four-legged animal or like you want to crawl. Now stretch forward, lift the alternative arm and leg, and stretch it straight.

20.   Prone canoe Pose:

This is one of the multi-advantageous postures because this is helpful in pain relieving as well as works very well when it comes to weight loss. Here you need to put both your hands straight while lying prone. Now lift the legs straight and together up and breathe well. Make sure you are not pressuring your hands. This boosts metabolism due to which fat formation is prevented and is also helpful for indigestion.

21.   Lizard Pose: The lizard pose is very helpful in releasing stress, fatigue, and tension.

This pose sure looks complicated but is not so. You can do this to relax your body after a hard day of work. It is instantly effective and very, very calming for the body.

The above stretches are a therapy for the mind and body as we already know and are very helpful. Keep breathing throughout the stretches feeling your whole body being filled with fresh oxygen as you breathe in rejuvenating your whole body and healing it when you exhale feel all the toxins coming out, and your body getting rid of unwanted dead cells, fat being melted away and your body getting toned and sculpted. Feel your mind and body relax as you finish each stretch and rest for a few seconds before starting the next stretch.

Conclusion: You can do these stretches after a warm-up, during an exercise segment, or after a workout segment. You must keep your mind focused on your body and on your breathing. in a calm manner. You can also do only stretches as a total workout by holding each pose initially for 10 seconds and as the days progress increase to 30 seconds then one or two minutes.

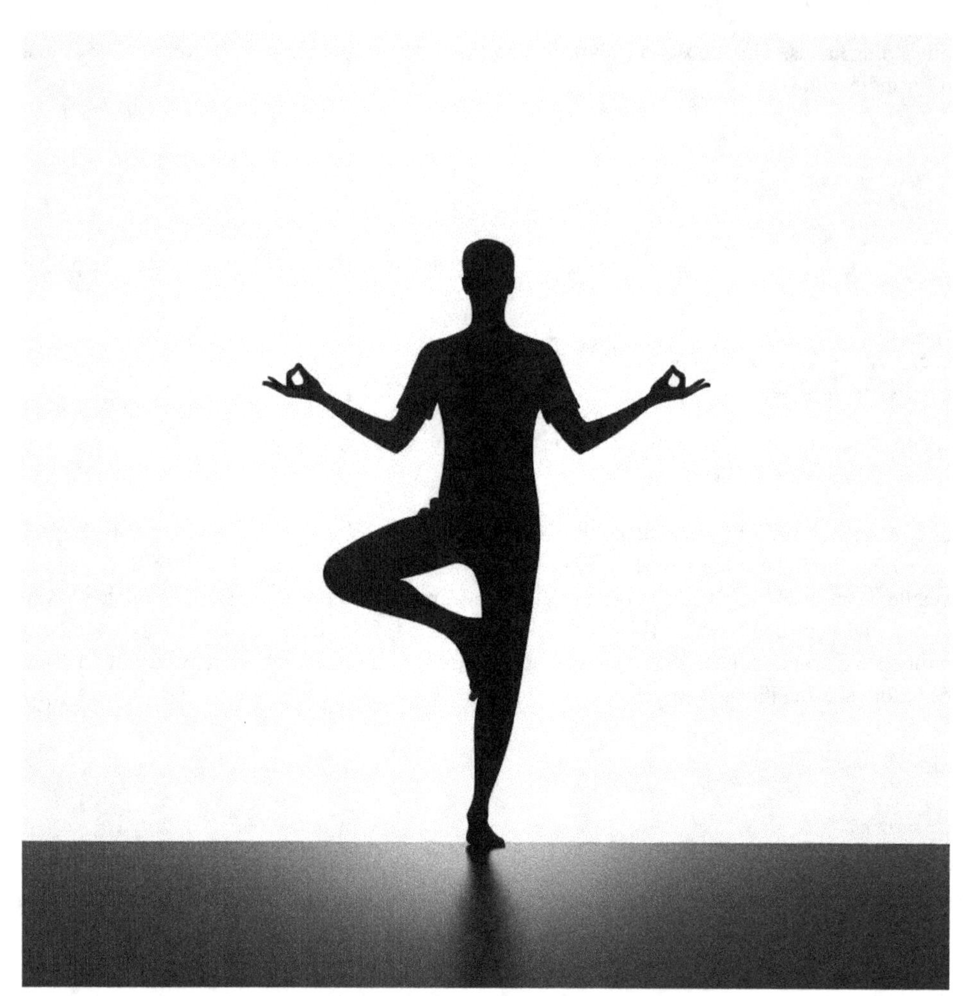

CHAPTER 7

WEIGHT MANAGEMENT AND NUTRITION

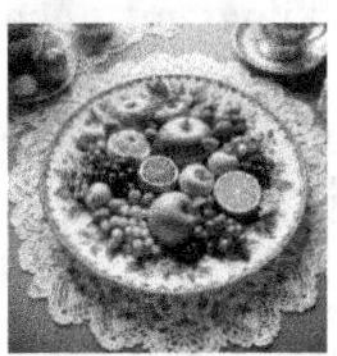

Physical activity and diet work together for better health. For example, physical activity increases the number of calories you burn. For those who have intentionally lost weight, being active makes it easier to maintain weight loss.

Combining exercise with a healthy diet is a more effective way to lose weight than depending on calorie restriction alone. Exercise can prevent or even reverse the effects of certain diseases. Exercise lowers blood pressure and cholesterol, which may prevent a heart attack. In addition, if you exercise, you lower your risk of developing certain types of cancers such as colon and breast cancer. Exercise is also known to help contribute to a sense of confidence and well-being, thus possibly lowering rates of anxiety and depression.

Exercise is helpful for weight loss and maintaining weight loss. Exercise can increase metabolism, or how many calories you burn in a day. It can also help you maintain and increase lean body mass, which also helps increase the number of calories you burn each day.

Lifestyle modification should be the central focus of any weight loss or weight maintenance program. Implementing a plan consisting of a reasonable dietary intake coupled with daily physical activity has been consistently shown to optimize weight loss and reduce the risk of disease.

If we look at the **causes and health complications of being overweight and obesity, we realize that it's the imbalance between energy intake and energy output that leads to excess accumulation of fat in various parts of the body which may impair our health.**
Body mass index (BMI) is a simple index of weight-for-height that is commonly used to classify overweight and obesity in adults. It is defined as a person's weight in kilograms divided by the square of his height in meters (kg/m^2).

Adults: For adults, WHO defines overweight as **a BMI** (Basic metabolic index) greater than or equal to 25 and obesity is a BMI greater than or equal to 30.

BMI provides the most useful population-level measure of overweight and obesity as it is the same for both sexes and all ages of adults. However, it should be considered a rough guide because it may not correspond to the same degree of fatness in different individuals.
For children, age needs to be considered when defining overweight and obesity. Overweight and obesity are linked to more deaths worldwide than underweight. Globally more people are obese than underweight – this occurs in every region except parts of sub-Saharan Africa and Asia.

The fundamental cause of obesity and overweight is an energy imbalance between calories consumed and calories expended. Globally, there has been an increased intake of energy-dense foods that are high in fat; and an increase in physical inactivity due to the increasingly sedentary nature of many forms of work, changing modes of transportation, and increasing urbanization. Changes in dietary and physical activity patterns are often the result of environmental and societal changes associated with development and lack of supportive policies in sectors such as health, agriculture, transport, urban planning, environment, food processing, distribution, marketing, and education.

There are many common health consequences of being overweight and obese. Raised BMI is a major risk factor for diseases such as cardiovascular diseases (mainly heart disease and stroke), which were the leading cause of death in 2012; diabetes; musculoskeletal disorders (especially osteoarthritis – a highly disabling degenerative disease of the joints); some cancers (including endometrial, breast, ovarian, prostate, liver, gallbladder, kidney, and colon).

The risk for these diseases increases, with increases in BMI.

Childhood obesity is associated with a higher chance of obesity, premature death, and disability in adulthood. But in addition to increased future risks, obese children experience breathing difficulties, increased risk of fractures, hypertension, early markers of cardiovascular disease, insulin resistance, and psychological effects.

Many people can also develop **psychological problems** because of being overweight or obese. For example: low self-esteem; poor self-image (not liking how you look); low confidence; and feelings of isolation. These feelings may affect your relationships with family members and friends and, if they become severe, may lead to depression.

Let's look at how overweight and obesity can be reduced. **Overweight and obesity,** as well as their related diseases, are largely preventable. Supportive environments and communities are fundamental in shaping people's choices, by making healthier foods and regular physical activity the easiest choice (the choice that is the most accessible, available, and affordable), and therefore preventing overweight and obesity.

There is no clear definition of a desirable or ideal body weight. Body weight for a given height of a person with good health and long lifespan is considered Ideal body weight. A much simpler and more acceptable measure is the ratio of weight and height, which estimates total body mass and correlates highly with the % of body fat.

The most commonly used ratio is the **BMI**. It is computed by dividing the weight in kilograms by the square of the height in meters *[BMI = Weight (kg) ÷ 2 (Height M)]*. The ideal ranges of weights for a given height are provided by WHO, which is useful for categorizing people as normal (ideal), undernourished, and overweight or obese in general, BMI ranging from 18.5 to 25 is considered to be normal. However, for Asians, it is recommended that the BMI should be between 18.5 and 23, since, they tend to have higher percentage body fat even at lower BMI compared to Caucasians and Europeans, which puts them at higher risk of chronic non-communicable diseases.

Are you obese or overweight? If you are obese or overweight, this means that you are carrying excess body fat. Being overweight or obese is not just about how you look. Over time, it means that you have an increased risk of developing various health problems. As an adult, you can find out whether you are overweight or obese and whether your health may be at risk, by calculating your body mass index (BMI) and measuring your waist circumference.

People are of different heights and build, so just weighing yourself cannot be used to decide if your weight is healthy. BMI (**Body mass index**) is used by healthcare professionals to assess if someone's weight is putting their health at risk. It is a measure of your weight related to your height.

To calculate your BMI, you divide your weight (in kilograms) by the square of your height (in meters). So, for example, if you weigh 70 kg and are 1.75 meters tall, your BMI is 70/(1.75 x 1.75), which is 22.9.

If you do not have scales at home, your practice nurse can measure your height, weigh you, and calculate your BMI.

There are different categories of obesity as follows:

- Ideal (normal) BMI is 18.5 to 24.9 kg/m2.

- A BMI of 25-29.9 kg/m2 is overweight.

- A BMI of 30-34.9 kg/m2 is obese (Grade I).

- A BMI of 35-39.9 kg/m2 is obese (Grade II).

- A BMI of $\geq$40 kg/m2 is obese (Grade III) or morbidly obese.

The more overweight you are, the more the risk to your health. For those who are obese (Grade III), weight is a serious and imminent threat to health. However, for those who are overweight or obese (Grade I), waist circumference is also taken into account to calculate the health risk.

Overall, BMI is a good estimate of how much of your body is made up of fat. However, BMI may be less accurate in very muscular people. This is because muscle weighs heavier than fat. So, someone who is very muscular may have a relatively high BMI due to the weight of their muscle bulk but have a proportionally low and healthy amount of body fat. Health risks are also calculated differently in older people.

Waist circumference is another way of assessing how healthy you are. More than a general accumulation, the distribution of fat around the abdomen is now considered to be more harmful than fat around the hips. Accumulation of fat around the abdomen indicated by higher waist circumference is considered a risk factor.

If you are overweight, measuring your waist circumference can also give some information about your risk of developing health problems (particularly coronary heart disease and type 2 diabetes). If two overweight or obese people have the same BMI, the person with a bigger waist circumference will be at a greater risk of developing health problems due to their weight. This is because it is not just *whether* you are carrying excess fat but *where* you are carrying it. The risks to your health are greater if you mainly carry a lot of extra fat around your waist ('apple-shaped'), rather than mainly on your hips and thighs ('pear-shaped').

The easiest way to measure your waist circumference is to place the tape measure around your waist at the belly button level.

As a rule for a man, if you have a waist measurement of 94 cm or above, the risk to your health is increased. If you have a waist measurement of 102 cm or above, the risk is even higher.

Similarly for a woman, if you have a waist measurement of 80 cm or above, the risk to your health is increased. If you have a waist measurement of 88 cm or above, the risk is even higher.

For people who are overweight, or obese (Grade 1), waist circumference is considered with BMI when assessing health risk. If you have a very high waist circumference, you may have a very high level of risk to your health even at the lower grades of obesity. If you have other medical conditions such as diabetes, high blood pressure, high cholesterol levels, or coronary heart disease, your risks are even higher. Weight loss is even more crucial.

Therefore, Diet and exercise play an important role in weight management. It is necessary to maintain desirable body weight by consuming just enough calories or adjusting physical activity to maintain energy balance *(intake = output)*. Body weight must, therefore, be checked and monitored periodically.

Several studies have suggested that hours spent watching television are strongly associated with weight gain in childhood and adolescence, mostly due to sedentary behavior, the tendency to consume snack foods while watching television, and the influence of the advertisements of energy-dense foods. Adults usually tend to gain weight between the ages of 25-50 years. In women, obesity develops just around pregnancy and after menopause.

As a result of a greater understanding of the effect of obesity on disease states, the emphasis for obesity treatment has dramatically shifted from weight management alone to a comprehensive program of lifestyle modification to decrease disease risk and enhance quality of life. **Lifestyle modification involves changes in dietary intake, physical activity, and behavior. Ideally, the appropriate treatment of obesity involves all of these components.**

Conclusion: Thanks to recent observational studies of men and women who have successfully lost weight and maintained that loss over a significant amount of time, it is now clear that lifestyle modification is the key to successful weight loss in the long term. Today, we must be aware that for optimal weight and disease management, **both dietary intake as well as exercise must be considered, along with behavioral therapy**, in the current therapeutic approaches to obesity. Ongoing research supports this recommendation. Several weight loss studies conducted on thousands of men and women found that their long-term success was due to a combination of a healthy, low-fat diet and regular, moderate exercise.

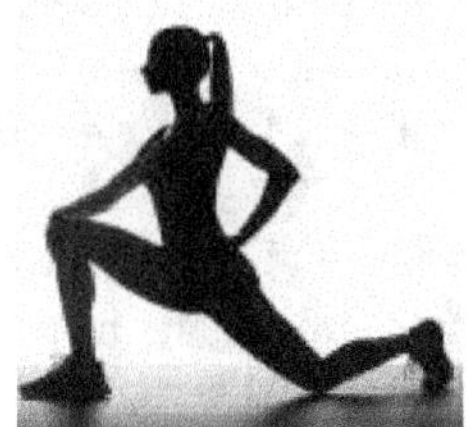

DIETARY INTAKE

An appropriate dietary management strategy should begin with a basic understanding of the interrelationship between calories ingested and expended. The critical balance between energy intake and energy expenditure determines body weight. The goal is to manipulate lifestyle through eating and exercise so that the obese individual's energy balance is negative over 24 hours. This means he or she has expended more calories than ingested. This can be achieved by: (1) decreasing food intake and keeping physical activity constant; (2) keeping food intake constant and increasing physical activity; or (3) decreasing food intake and increasing physical activity simultaneously.

Once you are a full-grown adult and have finished growing to your optimum height, the only way you can grow is sideways if you do not burn the calories you are consuming daily. The secret is to stop eating when your stomach is half full. Scientific studies have shown that it takes the body approximately 20 minutes to send the message to the brain that you are full and by that time you have already eaten so much more. **You can change this**. Imagine that your stomach is a circle, divide it into 4 quarters. Two parts for food, one part for water, and one part for air. This is the combination required for proper digestion. So when you have your meal you need to **stop when you are half full.**

Very-Low-Calorie Diets: In the past, most emphasis was placed on the first option. That is, the number of calories ingested formed the focal point of weight loss programs. Total fasts, in which less than 200 calories were ingested in 24 hours, had been used for quick weight loss. This type of program was harmful to the individual's lean body mass, which was consumed along with fat to maintain life.[6] Very-low-calorie diets (VLCDs) provide between 200 to 800 calories of daily food, often in the form of liquid commercial preparations. VLCDs were characterized by low compliance, medical complications, as well as poor long-term success once the individual resumed normal eating.[7]

Fad Diets are Nutritionally unbalanced. Today, the current consensus among nutrition scientists is that a balanced low-fat diet in combination with regular physical activity is the recommended approach to weight loss and maintenance. The Table summarizes the main characteristics of an appropriate and healthy dietary intake.

Total Calories	Women: no less than 1200 calories/day Men: no less than 1500 calories/day
Fat	30% of calories or less, reducing levels of saturated and trans fatty acids
Protein	20% to 25% of calories, averaging no less than 75 g/day
Carbohydrates	50% of calories, no less than 5 servings of fruits and vegetables daily Minimizing the ingestion of processed simple (table sugar) and complex (starches) sugars
Dietary Fiber	20-30 g/day from food sources
Water	No less than 1 liter per day
Alcohol	Limited or none

Current fad diets generally do not adhere to this prescription. These diets are characterized by a significant imbalance of macronutrients that leads to a decrease in the total micronutrients essential for the maintenance of critical cellular biochemical processes. The fad diets often emphasize the need to manipulate specific food groups. From this notion emerged the development of high-protein, low carbohydrate, high-fat (ketogenic) diets. The resultant ketosis is purported to cause appetite suppression and successful long-term weight loss. This has not been proven. Moreover, there is substantial scientific evidence demonstrating that such fad diets are dangerous to health in the long run. Nausea, fatigue, postural hypotension, foul breath, high cholesterol content, elevated uric acid levels, and calcium loss have all been reported in individuals following these diets.

Conclusion: My concluding message is that once you are a full-grown adult and have finished growing to your optimum height, you will most probably grow more sideways (you know what I mean) if you do not burn those extra calories you are consuming daily. There is a tried-and-true solution to that. The secret to stop eating when your stomach is half full! You will give me that look saying will I not feel hungry faster? Well, the body does not need the additional intake unless you are going to use it by doing more activity. Hunger is most probably only in your mind so you need to distract your thoughts, by drinking water, coconut water, diluted lime juice, or a light buttermilk. This is because you have already consumed enough solids and that is sufficient for you! Scientific studies have shown that it takes the body approximately 20 minutes to send the message to the brain that you are full and by that time you have already eaten so much more!

I seriously suggest you do this. Take a pen or pencil and a sheet of paper. Draw a circle. Divide it into 4 quarters. Assuming the circle is our stomach, allocate two-quarters of it for food, one part for water, and one part for air. This is the combination required for proper digestion. Put up this poster where you can see it every day.

Eat healthy, exercise, be active, sleep for at least 7 hours every night, make sure your bowels are working regularly and have a positive attitude towards Life. You only live once. Be fit to live it to the full. Wishing you a high quality of life. **Cheers!**

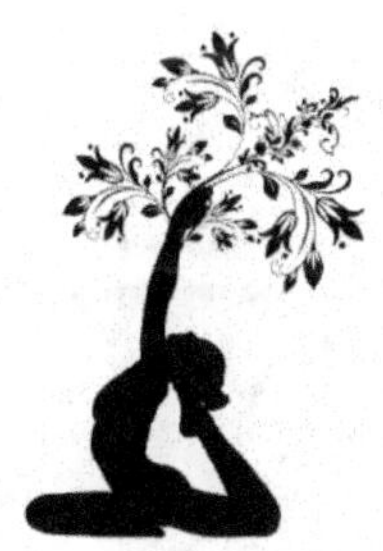

RESOURCES, LINKS, and RECOMMENDED READINGS

Wardlaw, Smith. Contemporary Nutrition: A Functional Approach. 2nd ed: 2012. McGraw Hill.

Williams Melvin. Nutrition for health, fitness and sports. 2004.Mc Graw Hill

Joshi AS. Nutrition and Dietetics 2010. Tata Mc Graw Hill

Centers for Disease Control and Prevention. U.S. Obesity Trends. 2011. Available at: http

Artificial intelligence

McArdle WD, Katch FI, Katch VL. Exercise Physiology: Energy, Nutrition, and Human Performance. Philadelphia, Pa: Lea and Febiger; 1981.

AFAA - Textbook of Aerobics and Fitness Association of

America Various textbooks on Yoga https://www.healthline.com

Chinese Body Clock: About, Benefits, Research (healthline.com)

YouTube: https://youtube.com/@charmainecpaul

CONGRATULATIONS ON TAKING A STEP TOWARDS GREAT HEALTH AND FITNESS

IF YOU LIKED THE BOOK KINDLY LEAVE A REVIEW. THANK YOU

Upcoming books

1) YOGA - Disease Prevention and Control

2) MERIDIAN WISDOM - Acupuncture and Naturopathy for good health